DON'T LET SUGAR SUCK YOU IN

DO NOT ALLOW YOURSELF TO BE LET.

BY

KING ADAM

TABLE OF CONTENT

Introduction

Given that many people consume more sugar than is ideal for health, the issue of excess sugar and its effects on health is crucial. Sugar is a type of carbohydrate that is added to many processed and packaged foods and drinks in addition to occurring naturally in some foods, such as fruits and vegetables. While a healthy diet can contain small amounts of sugar, excessive sugar consumption can be harmful to your health. Excessive sugar consumption has been associated with a higher risk of weight gain, chronic diseases like type 2 diabetes, heart disease, and obesity, as well as dental issues. The mood and energy levels can also change after consuming large amounts of sugar. It is crucial to be conscious of how much sugar you are consuming and to make decisions that will help prevent or reduce excessive sugar intake..

Chapter 1 varieties of sugar

There are several varieties of sugar that are frequently consumed. Others are added to foods and beverages to sweeten them while some are naturally occurring. Here is a quick breakdown of the various sugar varieties.

Coca leaves have been consumed for centuries as chewing tobacco and for making tea. Nothing was wrong, and everything was as it should be. But after that, they underwent arduous processing to become cocaine, a dangerous and addictive substance. Same thing happened to the helpless poppy flower. Before becoming a potent, dangerous, and addictive opiate, tea was a useful and safe substance that was frequently consumed for pain relief and relaxation. But it became excessively processed.

Glucose: Grains, fruits, and vegetables all contain simple sugars like glucose. It is used by cells to make ATP, the body's primary energy source, which is then utilized by the body.

Fruits, vegetables, and honey all contain the simple sugar fructose. It is also used as an additional sweetener in a lot of processed foods and drinks.

A sugar called lactose is found in milk and other dairy products. It is broken down in the body by the enzyme lactase. Galactose and glucose make up its structure.

Sucrose: The disaccharide sugar known as sucrose is created when glucose and fructose combine. High fructose corn syrup (HFCS), which is more commonly known as table sugar . fructose-rich corn syrup, is made from corn starch and is used to sweeten foods and beverages. Processed foods and beverages frequently use it because it is less expensive than sugar and easier to incorporate into products.

Maltodextrin: Maltodextrin is a carbohydrate made from the starches of corn, rice, or potatoes. It is regularly used as a filler or thickener in processed foods and beverages.

Chapter 2 What sugar does to your body

There are many ways that eating too much sugar can be bad for your health. While a small amount of added sugars can be included in a balanced diet, consuming large amounts of them can have negative effects on your physical and mental health. The health effects of excessive sugar consumption are listed below, along with some potential symptoms.

An increased risk of tooth decay is one of the most well-known consequences of consuming too much sugar. The enamel of the teeth can be eroded by the acid that the bacteria in the mouth produce as they consume sugars. Cavities may result from this, which may aggravate the sensitivity and pain of the teeth.

Obesity and weight gain are both influenced by excessive sugar consumption. Sugar contains a lot of calories, and it's simple to eat more than you need without realizing it. Your body stores excess calories as fat if you consume more calories than you burn off. Particularly if you aren't exercising, this may result in weight gain. Risk of type 2 diabetes rising: A diet high in sugar can raise the possibility of getting the disease. The glucose that is produced when you eat sugar is then released into the bloodstream by your body. As a result, the pancreas secretes insulin, which aids in controlling blood sugar levels. If you eat too much sugar, your body may develop insulin resistance, which can result in high blood sugar levels and a higher risk of developing diabetes.

Heart disease risk is raised by consuming too much sugar. The risk of cardiovascular disease is increased by high blood sugar levels, which can harm blood vessels. Large sugar intake can also raise blood levels of bad cholesterol, which can raise the risk of heart disease even more.

Increased risk of non-alcoholic fatty liver disease: Eating a lot of sugar can result in an accumulation of fat in the liver, which can raise the risk of non-alcoholic fatty liver disease. A buildup of fat in the liver cells is the defining feature of this condition, which can cause liver injury and scarring.

A lot of sugar consumption can cause blood sugar fluctuations, which can alter mood and energy levels. You may experience a brief surge of energy after eating sugar because it causes your blood sugar levels to rise quickly. However, you might feel exhausted and agitated as your blood sugar levels fall.

Acne and other skin issues are more likely to occur when a person consumes too much sugar. An increase in oil production and inflammation may result from sugar's impact on the body's hormone production. Other skin conditions, such as acne, may also develop as a result of this.

Immune system deterioration: A diet rich in sugar can impair immunity, making it more difficult for the body to fend off infections and diseases. Large sugar intake can affect how well white blood cells, which are in charge of warding off infections, function.

Mineral Balance: If you have trouble sleeping at night, experience constipation, or experience other problems, your mineral balance may be out of whack. If you eat a lot of sugar, you might have depleted all of your magnesium stores. More chromium will also be lost through your urine if you consume a lot of sugar.

Behavior Issues: As any parent on the planet will attest, sugar, as well as a lack of it, can have an effect on a child's behavior. If a child is hungry and their blood sugar is low, they will be cranky and sleepy. A child who consumes too much sugar will become agitated and animated. A healthy blood sugar level is essential for better behavior. Triglycerides in the blood are elevated for several reasons, none of which manifest as symptoms. You cannot tell if you have high triglycerides without a blood test. It is typically a part of your complete cholesterol test.

Chapter 3 The Unexpected Locations Sugar Hides

It can be difficult to identify the sugar that is hidden in our diet. You'll be shocked at how many products contain extra, frequently unnecessary sugar.

Breakfast cereal Contrary to what the majority of you might have assumed, we are not talking about the sugar in sugary cereal. Sugar is concealed in cereals that are advertised as being healthy. Some "healthy" cereals contain more than 23 grams of sugar.

•**Asian Food** - Most Asian food sold in stores or packaged in products has a significant sugar content. even sushi. The sushi rice preparation procedure includes the use of sugar. To ensure that the sugar content isn't too high, make your own Asian food.

Thankfully, reading soup and sauce labels on cans and packages is all that is required. Even spaghetti sauce and gravy can occasionally have higher sugar content than soda, with some yogurts having more than 15 grams of sugar. If you want to be certain to eat less sugar, read labels, look for products with no added sugar, or make your own.

• **Frozen yogurt**: Just because something contains the word "yogurt," doesn't automatically make it healthy. It is equivalent to regular ice cream in terms of sugar content. indeed, dessert. A dessert-like strategy ought to be used. Don't consider it a meal and only eat it as a snack. It won't make you healthier. Since the amount of sugar in either is the same, you are now free to switch to real ice cream if you prefer it.

• **Smoothies:** Taking advantage of their popularity, there are many smoothie shops around. However, most smoothie shops use fruit to which sugar has been added, negating any benefits that drinking a smoothie might have. If you make your own dried fruit, be careful when recipes call for it. Fresh, whole fruit is always preferred.

• **Bread:** While some types of bread are nutritious, most are made with sugar and highly refined flour. These two affect blood sugar levels. Reading the labels is crucial because even wheat bread can have a lot of sugar in it. Typically, the sugar content of rye or spelt bread is low. Making your own is another option if you want to avoid unhealthy additives and sugar.

• **Condiments:** We all like drizzling everything in sauce, right? If, however, you accidentally dip your celery or apples, you might be making matters worse. Examine the condiment labels or create your own at home. Low-sugar ketchup is just one of the many condiments that are readily available today.

• Canned beans: When buying beans in a can, always read the label, especially if the beans have any kind of sauce on them, like baked beans or chili beans. Most of the time, they are so sweet that if you compared them to cakes, you couldn't tell which was which based solely on the sugar content.

- **Muffins:** Despite the fact that you are probably already aware that some muffins are high in sugar, even those that sound healthy are really just cakes disguised as muffins with healthy ingredients. Each one is incredibly sweet. But you can find some recipes for low-sugar muffins online; just do a search. No need to go without exists for you.

- **Yogurt:** Like frozen yogurt, the majority of sweetened yogurt, including low-fat yogurt, is high in sugar. The best solution for this problem is to make your own yogurt or to eat it as a dessert. You can also buy plain yogurt and mix in your own fruit and stevia to make a low-sugar snack that is healthy because of the probiotics in yogurt. The key takeaway is that anything that has been prepared and packaged might have too much sugar. Reading the labels and forming your own opinions are preferable. Don't forget that 90 grams of added sugar per day—or 5% of total calories—is the upper limit for adult intake.

.

Chapter 4 What Amount of Sugar Is Too Much

The difference between sugar that occurs naturally and sugar that is added must be understood. Although plant food is good for you, it contains sugar. In fact, a sizable portion of your plate should be made up of plant-based foods if you want to be as healthy as possible.

Adults should keep their daily sugar intake to a maximum of 90 grams, according to the study's findings. You can calculate how much of that is added sugar based on your ideal daily caloric intake. In other words, 90 grams of sugar are acceptable if you consume 1500 calories per day. You get to choose how much of that gets processed and given more sugar. The less added sugar you consume, the better for your health. You can therefore take some chances with your health and enjoy yourself on your birthday. Realizing that a cup of grapes contains 15 grams of sugar while a can of coke contains 39 grams makes the choice easier. A sugar-free Zevia or, even better, a LaCroix might be appropriate if you're really thirsty. But a cup of grapes and a tall glass of filtered water will keep you fuller for longer. Finding sugar substitutes that you genuinely like and enjoy while staying under your daily limit of 90 grams is crucial. The more natural sugars within those 90 grams you consume, the better you'll feel. They are generally quite low. glycemic options   available   to   you.

Fruit

 Apples – 1 small = 15g
pricots – 1 cup = 15g
Banana – 1 medium = 14g
Blackberries – 1 cup whole = 7g
Blueberries – 1 cup whole = 15g
Cantaloupe – 1 cup diced = 12g
Cranberries – 1 cup whole = 4g
Grapefruit – 1 cup = 16g
Guavas – 1 cup = 15g
Honeydew – 1 cup diced = 14g
Lemons – 1 wedge = 0.2g
Limes - 1 wedge = 0.15g
Papaya – 1 cup 1" cubed = 11g
Peaches – 1 cup sliced = 13g
 Raspberries – 1 cup whole = 5g
Rhubarb – 1 cup diced = 1.3g
Strawberries – 1 cup whole = 7g
Tomatoes – 1 large whole = 4.8g
Watermelon – 1 cup diced = 9g

Vegetables

Artichokes – 1 large = 1.6g
Asparagus – 1 cup = 2.5g
Broccoli – 1 cup chopped = 1.5g
Carrots – 1 medium = 2.9g

Celery – 1 cup chopped = 1.8g
Corn – 1 cup = 1.1g
Cucumber – 1 8-in = 5g
Green Beans – 1 cup = 3.3g
Kale – 1 cup chopped = 1.6g
Lettuce – 1 head = 2.8g

Soybean sprouts – 1 cup = 0.1g
Spinach – 1 cup = 0.1g
Summer squash – 1 cup sliced = 2.5g
Swiss chard – 1 cup = 0.4g

The majority of natural foods, as you can see, don't actually contain "too much" sugar. You'll be surprised at how much you can eat if you stay away from added sugars if you can consume 90 grams of sugar per day and choose wisely from the lower sugar fruits and vegetables. You can choose what to eat in every circumstance when you take into account that one teaspoon of processed sugar contains 4 points 2 grams.

Chapter 5 Are You Addicted to Sugar?

Be aware that your daily intake of carbohydrates has nothing to do with the 90 grams of sugar that you are permitted to consume per UK government guidelines. You must keep track of this distinct number.

Here are a few typical actions that indicate a sugar addition.

If there are certain foods that you simply cannot stop eating, assume that they are likely high in sugar. Since sugar doesn't actually fill you up, it's challenging to stop eating it.

The situation worsens when sugar, sodium, and fat are combined. For instance, you may be consuming donuts that are high in fat and salt as well, but it is unlikely that you would consume them if they were devoid of sugar.

You Have a Craving for Processed Carbs: If you have a constant craving for processed carbohydrates like chips, crackers, and bread, you may only have a sugar addiction. Over time, cutting out added sugars can frequently reduce your cravings for highly processed carbohydrates.

Salt and sugar pair well in processed foods, which is why you crave salty foods. If you believe that all it would take to make you happy is to lick a salt lick, you may be addicted to sugar. Check the sugar content of the snacks you typically eat. If they have been heavily processed, you can be certain that they have too much added sugar.

You Want Meat: Although it might seem strange, if you crave meat but don't actually need it or aren't actually that When you're hungry, you might actually be yearning for the spices that are frequently served with meat, such as wing sauce, which is very sweet.

The maximum recommended daily intake of sugar is 90 grams, so consider whether your typical meal exceeds this amount. This does not mean you should consume that much sugar. If you begin to feel unwell or unhealthy, you can always lower that amount. The best way to achieve this is to consume fewer added sugars and to stick to naturally occurring sugar that is derived from plants.

Sugar May Be the Cause of Your Persistent Moodiness and Grumpiness You Get Moody Without Sugar. If your blood sugar fluctuates frequently throughout the day, you may become irritable when it drops. This can get worse if you consume sugary foods like candy, which cause you to jump and fall quickly.

Long-day workers—students in particular—often experience this. You Feel Powerless Over Sugar: Do you ever feel like you don't even want to eat a sugary snack when you know it will cheer you up? While consuming a sugary snack will temporarily help, you'd be better off selecting a fruit snack that contains only natural sugars and fiber to help slow the rate of sugar absorption.

Look back on the entire day. You Start and End Your Day with Sugar. What do you eat for breakfast, what do you eat before bed, what do you eat every morning and every evening? If you eat sugar in the morning and at night, especially added processed sugar rather than sugar from whole plants, this may be a sign of a sugar addiction.

Chapter 6 How to Fight Sugar Addiction Withdrawal Symptoms

You're going to experience withdrawal symptoms when you first begin eliminating added sugar from your diet, especially if some of your sweet treats contained caffeine. Since you don't want to consume a lot of artificial sugar substitutes, it is best to attempt to treat each symptom you encounter.

Depression: If you notice that after cutting out added sugar you are feeling depressed, make sure you are eating some natural sugars, such as those found in fruit and vegetables. You do not want to have no carbohydrates. After consuming carbs, you feel good. No additional sugar, fat, or oil should be added when eating them.

Less caffeine consumption is the most likely cause of a headache. However, if you find that you are getting headaches, make sure you are properly hydrated. If you're accustomed to drinking sugary drinks, it can be difficult to drink plain water. However, it's important to make sure you get enough water each day.

Anxiety: Everyone has a unique way of experiencing anxiety. Fluttering in the stomach is a common symptom. Others experience rapid heartbeat or shortness of breath. Extreme severity may occur in some cases. The best course of action is to visit your doctor for a blood test if you notice that you're experiencing a lot of anxiety. Disorders like hypothyroidism, which have nothing to do with sugar restriction, can cause anxiety.

If not, just make sure you're drinking enough water, getting enough sleep, and eating enough calories to keep your weight at its ideal level.

You may experience an irritable mood if your blood sugar levels drop too low. To remedy this, eat more frequently. Try to balance the portions of protein, fat, and carbohydrates in your meals to meet your specific needs. You'll be more likely to become moody if you don't allow yourself to get too hungry. Have healthy snacks on hand, like apples and peanut butter without added sugar.

Fatigue: You're still experiencing the 3 o'clock slump. You may not be getting enough carbohydrates in your diet if you frequently feel fatigued and confused. Eat lots of vegetables because they are nutritious carbs. There's a chance that you should drink more water.

One of the earliest signs of dehydration is aching muscles. It can be difficult for many people who previously mainly drank sugary drinks to get enough water. Get eight or more glasses of water each day. Snack on hydrating foods like apples, carrots, oranges, and other fresh fruits and vegetables.

When you realize that you are experiencing intense sugar cravings, it is time to review your list of things to do when you are experiencing cravings. You can still indulge in something sweet, but opt for something natural rather than candy or processed foods, like a bowl of berries or thinly sliced apples. The symptoms of sugar withdrawal are more difficult to manage for some people than for others. Self-care necessitates endurance. If you cave and eat processed sugar, drink more water, increase your exercise, and be prepared the next time with a healthy snack. Don't forget to try the vinegar and greens as well.

Chapter 7 How to Avoid Sugar Cravings with These Recipes

One way to avoid consuming too much sugar is to be prepared. If you keep food on hand to eat when you're hungry, when you're tired, or when you have cravings, you'll do much better sticking to your goals.

Dessert of Frozen Fruit.

This is more of a concept than a specific recipe. A food processor, a high-speed blender, a magic bullet, or any of the aforementioned tools can be used. Yonana Frozen Healthy Dessert Maker is another option. The fruit you want to use in a while can simply be frozen, then blended in a blender, food processor, or put into a Yonana. Both the taste and the preparation are simple. Use the most ripe fruit you can find for the sweetest flavor.

Snacks The best snacks have a balanced protein to fat composition. These low-sugar snack ideas will be beneficial if you even slightly miss sugar.

Slice an apple and spread sugar-free peanut butter on top to replace bread with apples and peanut butter. The best peanut butter only contains one element. Peanuts. Because apples contain fiber, sugar digests more slowly as a result. Due to its high protein and fat content, peanut butter helps you stay full.

Fiber Rich Loaf

Everyone enjoys bread, but it can contain a lot of sugar. However, you can make your own nutritious, low-sugar bread that is high in fiber.

No Sugar Fiber Loaf

1 cup hulled, salt-free raw pumpkin seeds

1/2 cup hemp seeds

1/2 cup raw peeled almonds

1.5 cup rolled oats

2 tbsp chia seeds

3 tbsp psyllium husk powder

1 tsp fine grain sea salt

1 tbsp honey

3 tbsp apple sauce

1.5 cup water

assemble all of the dry ingredients. Setting aside. Mix the wet ingredients collectively in a different bowl. Then, combine the dry ingredients with the wet ones. Mix until a thick dough forms. If you decide it's too dry, more water can be added. After forming into a dough, put it in a bread pan. Your bread pan can be prepared in one of two ways: with parchment paper as a liner or by rubbing oil on it with a paper towel. Place the dough and pan in a warm area, covered, for at least two hours.

of the jar. applying a towel. If you lightly touch the dough with your finger, it will still hold its shape when the dough has sufficiently risen, which will allow you to know when it has. For about 30 to 40 minutes, bake on the middle rack in a 350°F oven. When a loaf of bread is finished, it will sound hollow.

vegetables that have undergone fermentation.

Let's make this simpler. Large quantities of vegetables can be pre-cut, or you can buy pre-chopped vegetables in bags or from the salad bar in the fresh section of your neighborhood grocery store. The course of action is up to you. But you should still cut them into smaller pieces. It's likely that pieces of 1/2 inch will function best.

A few glass jars with sealable lids, such as canning jars, are also necessary. Chop as many vegetables as you like. Include a few apples or carrots because of their sweet flavor. Add some ginger if you like the flavor. Salt should be used to season everything. Each jar of your vegetable mixture should be completely filled with your chopped vegetable mixture. Leave an inch of space at the top. Mash the vegetables and add them to the jar. They must firmly fit. Then, fill each jar with the next mixture until it is one inch below the top.

Brine .

4 cups of water.

1 teaspoon of sea salt.

Salt must be thoroughly dissolved in the mixture. Make sure the vegetable mixture in the jar is always submerged in water. If necessary, press the mixture down using a weight or stone. The covering is made out of cheesecloth and a rubber band. Maintain in a warm area for three to five days.

Every day, check the mixture to make sure everything is still submerged in brine. Your fermented vegetables will be ready when they begin to bubble. That proves that the fermentation process is complete. A pleasant, slightly sour aroma should emanate from your vegetables. They should be tasty as well. After that, secure the jars' regular lids before putting them in the refrigerator.

Avoiding added sugars is a good starting point if you're serious about overcoming your sugar cravings, improving your health, and losing weight. You shouldn't worry about the sugar that naturally occurs in the plants you eat, but you should try to limit the amount of extremely sweet fruit like dates and dried fruits.

Take each day as it comes. To avoid overindulging when you're hungry, remember to eat until you're satisfied. You'll quickly break your sugar habit if you drink enough water, exercise, and get enough sunlight.

Chapter 8 Advice on How to Kick the Sugar Habit

Thankfully, giving up your sugar addiction doesn't take much work. It's only challenging if you want to consume no sugar. That wouldn't be useful. Instead, start with a decrease and then steadily decrease it more and more through shrewd dietary decisions.

Avoid Processed Foods: Processed foods are the main source of added sugar in food. If processed food doesn't have a lot of sugar, it usually has a lot of chemicals. By avoiding processed foods, you can almost entirely eliminate the added sugar you consume.

Get Lots of Sunlight: Although it may seem strange, serotonin, the feel-good hormone, is one of the reasons why people enjoy eating sugar. If you eat a lot of sugar, your serotonin levels will rise. Naturally, you also have a crash. The sun is one of the better approaches that are available. Naturally, vitamin D will also be given to you because it is known to improve mood.

Sleep a lot: If you have trouble falling asleep at night, figure out what's causing it. Avoid sugar, caffeine, and anything stimulating two to three hours before going to bed. You should avoid carrying anything to bed in order to get the best sleep.

Drink Enough Water: It's critical to maintain hydration if you want to prevent cravings of any kind, including those for sugar. When you are born, your thirst detector is absolutely accurate. However, due to the stresses of life, we frequently disregard our bodies' signals. Therefore, weigh yourself before drinking to ensure that you consume at least 64 to 100 ounces of water each day.

Maintain a balanced blood sugar level by concentrating on stability. One way to do this is to eat at regular intervals. While some people only eat the customary three meals a day, you might eat six. It depends on what suits you the best. It is advisable to eat when you are truly hungry.

Eat more green vegetables like spinach, kale, turnip greens, and others to reduce your cravings for sweets. As a result, if you have a craving for something sweet, try eating some steamed spinach with good red wine vinegar on it. This will satisfy your craving. Include Fermented Foods and Drinks: Fermented foods and drinks are excellent at controlling your stomach's acid and bacteria as well as your cravings for sweets. You can buy prepared fermented foods or make your own. It's important to note that only a small amount of sugar is utilized during the fermentation process, but that's okay.

Meditate: The urge for sugar may occasionally be a sign that you need to take a moment to gather your thoughts and relax. The effects of anxiety on hunger and cravings are profound. A daily meditation session should last at least 10 minutes. You can try prayer or silent meditation if you don't want to meditate. Including these suggestions in your daily routine can be extremely helpful when trying to stop sugar cravings and break your sugar habit. Also remember that it won't occur immediately. Just focus on attracting more positive aspects of life rather than expelling negative ones.